Z. E. FARHADOVA

A Little Baby in the Family

Contents

1

Introduction

—A young woman should also know how to prepare for motherhood and care for a little one, Aunt Carla said with cunning in her voice.

—This is also an important topic, and I will listen with pleasure, because sooner or later it will affect me too," Natasha was delighted.

2

Are you planning a child?

The desire to have children — is a natural desire of a woman, but before you take this step, think carefully: are you ready for the birth of a baby?

Never decide to do this with the sole purpose of keeping your loved one or because all your friends already have children.

Remember: a child is a person whom you will be responsible for.

It all starts at conception

Conception occurs at the moment of fusion of female and male reproductive cells (egg and sperm). The egg is surrounded by a large number of sperm, but only one fertilizes it. Much less often, several male reproductive cells can penetrate the egg, then twins or triplets are born.

From the moment of fertilization, the egg becomes an egg in which cell division occurs.

About 10 days after fertilization, the egg descends into the uterus and implants into it, that is, it is implanted into the uterus. The embryo begins to actively develop.

3

Boy or girl

The sex of the child is determined at the moment of fertilization. With the help of ultrasound, you can determine already in the third month of pregnancy whether you will have a son or a daughter.

You can plan the gender of the child, taking into account the periods of renewal of the blood composition. Science has proven that a woman's blood composition is completely renewed once every three years, and a man's once every four years. The blood that is younger dominates. Consequently, if the mother's blood is younger, then a girl is born, if the father's blood dominates, then a boy is born. This method of planning the gender of the unborn child is effective in 80 cases out of 100.

A little about heredity

The laws of heredity were discovered back in the 19th century by Georg Mendel.

Research has shown that the chromosomes contained in the cell are responsible for heredity. Each cell includes 44 ordinary chromosomes and 2 sex chromosomes.

Ovum: 44 + 2 (XX)

Sperm: 44 + 2 (XV)

After fertilization, chromosome division occurs.

Ovum: 44 + XX division process 22 + X

Spermatozoon: 44 + XV division process 22 + X or 22 + V

As you understand, a complete set of chromosomes is formed in a new cell, one half of which carries the hereditary characteristics of the mother, and the other of the father. Chromosomes are arranged in pairs. They contain tiny particles of genes. Maternal and paternal genes are always located nearby. In this regard, the future baby will look like both mom and dad.

4

Waiting for a baby

Expecting a child is one of the most important periods of your life. After all, the well-being of the unborn baby largely depends on how the pregnancy goes. Keep in mind that pregnancy is a completely natural state for a woman; nature makes sure that you give birth to a child without any complications.

Signs of pregnancy:
1. Stopping menstruation.
2. Enlargement of the mammary glands, slight tingling in them.
3. Darkening of the nipples and halos around them.
4. Formation of new glands near the nipple.
5. Release of colostrum during compression of the mammary gland.
6. The vaginal mucosa becomes darker in color.
7. Enlarged uterus.
8. Feeling of nausea.
9. Change in taste preferences.

If you find these signs, then you definitely need to undergo a gynecological examination, and if pregnancy is confirmed, register with a antenatal clinic and enroll in courses for expectant mothers.

Pregnancy lasts on average 280 days, in other words 40 weeks, 10 lunar or 9 calendar months. The date of birth is determined as follows: 7 days are added to the first day of the last menstruation and 3 months are subtracted. So, if the last day of menstruation fell on October 20, then add 7 to 20 (20+7=27), and now from October 27, count back 3 months (October, September, August), we get July, This means the baby will be born around July 27th.

Greater accuracy is obtained by ultrasound examination and determination of how enlarged the uterus is.

So, you're pregnant. During this period, a number of changes occur in your body, which helps create the necessary conditions for the development of a healthy child. You must ensure that nothing from the outside has a detrimental effect on your body.

5

Personal hygiene of the expectant mother

During pregnancy, take special care of yourself and follow the rules of hygiene.

A woman who is expecting a child must take a cool shower every day. The water temperature should not exceed 35 degrees (95 degrees fahrenheit). The body is washed with soap, it is best to use baby soap, and wipe with a terry towel. For washing, use warm boiled water; douching is avoided. You should wash yourself at least 3 times a day.

If you prefer a bath, then it is better for you not to overuse visits to the steam room, because this can have a detrimental effect on pregnancy.

Also, you should not take very hot baths, as they cause fatigue and become overly relaxing.

In principle, taking baths is not contraindicated, but to avoid accidents, the bottom of the bath should be covered.

For the same purpose, you can place a small bench at the bottom of the bath and wash while sitting on it.

Please note that swimming in the river is not prohibited, and sea swimming is not recommended, as the sea is quite rough. You should not swim far from the shore, because during pregnancy the likelihood of cramps increases.

Nails are cut short during pregnancy, this reduces the possibility of contact with infections.

It is important to brush your teeth regularly, and in case of disease, promptly seek help from a dentist. Everything you use during pregnancy should be strictly individual. Avoid any contact with sick people.

6

Clothes and shoes of the expectant mother

Clothes also require close attention. It should be comfortable and not put pressure on the stomach.

As for underwear, it should be changed daily.

It is important to carefully select bras during pregnancy, taking into account that during this period the mammary glands enlarge. The bra should be wide enough and not constrict the chest. It is better to use a bra with its clasp located in the front.

It is recommended to wear panties only in the warm season; in winter, insulated leggings that do not tighten the hips and stomach are more suitable.

From the sixth month of pregnancy, it is recommended to support the abdomen with a bandage that prevents the skin from stretching. It is better to sew dresses with a loose, non-fitted cut.

As for a pregnant woman's shoes, they should have low, stable heels and be comfortable.

7

About walks and trips

The expectant mother should take walks every day (except in cases where the doctor recommended complete rest).

In total, you need to be in the fresh air for at least 3 hours a day.

If possible, you should spend more time outside the city.

It is strictly forbidden to ride a motorcycle.

You can drive a car on your own until the seventh month of pregnancy. Then, due to the enlargement of the abdomen and the weakening of the reaction, this should be abandoned.

In the last months of pregnancy, it is not recommended to take long trips by train, much less fly by plane.

8

Nutrition and sleep

Now that you are expecting a child, you should pay even more attention to your nutrition, because your body's metabolism is accelerating. You may have to give up some foods, such as pork, fried potatoes, pistachios, that is, products that contain excessive amounts of fat or starch.

You should also reduce your intake of liquids to prevent swelling.

Drink tea and coffee containing caffeine in limited quantities.

You can drink good white wine in small doses, but you need to quit smoking.

Your daily menu should include foods containing large amounts of protein: milk, cheese, cottage cheese, lean meat, fish, eggs.

Also, do not forget to include vegetables and fruits, and wholemeal bread in your diet. These products normalize intestinal function and contain vitamins.

It is vitamins that help strengthen the immune system.

Vitamin A prevents the occurrence of visual impairment and skin diseases. It is found in green onions, carrots, milk, and fish oil.

B vitamins stimulate the work- capacity, appetite, reduce the possibility of edema. They can be obtained by eating meat, spinach, and oatmeal.

Vitamin C is responsible for the body's resistance to disease. It is contained in black currants, lemons, and rosehips.

Vitamin D activates the general condition of the body. It is found in fish oil, liver, and egg yolk. Under the influence of sunlight, it is produced by the body itself,

While expecting a child, a woman's body requires a large amount of iron (up to 20 mg per day). Yolks, prunes, and pomegranates contain iron.

Please note that a pregnant woman needs to reduce her salt intake to 5 mg per day.

You should not overuse sweet and flour foods. It is advisable to get carbohydrates from fresh vegetables and fruits.

Eat regularly, often enough, but remember that the food should not be too high in calories.

If you have an incorrect diet during pregnancy, you may develop a tendency to constipation. The functioning of the gastrointestinal tract needs to be stabilized. To do this, you should drink water with honey dissolved in it in the morning, and have breakfast with oatmeal and fruit. Fruits should also be included in dinner.

Remember: laxative medications are used only after consultation with an obstetrician-gynecologist, as these medications can cause miscarriage.

And now about your sleep: you should sleep at least 8 hours a day. You should not sleep for a long time during the day, because such rest can cause insomnia at night. It is recommended to rest quietly in the afternoon.

9

About physical education

A woman who goes in for sports endures pregnancy and childbirth more easily. Of course, if you are involved in pole vaulting, horse riding or water skiing, then it is better to give up these activities during this period. However, a pregnant woman is not prohibited from going to the mountains if she can avoid lifting heavy equipment, swimming short distances.

Gymnastics is of paramount importance in terms of preparing for childbirth. Physical exercise improves well-being, strengthens the abdominal muscles, and prevents complications during childbirth and the postpartum period.

Remember: the set of exercises must be agreed upon with your doctor.

Each exercise is performed for no longer than 3 minutes, followed by a pause of 30 seconds. You need to exercise for 20-25 minutes every day. Before performing the exercises, do not forget to ventilate the room, get rid of the bra that restricts movement, take off your shoes, and take off your glasses.

It is better to practice on the floor with a carpet or blanket.

It's good if you do gymnastics to music.

Here are exercises you can do after consulting your doctor.

1. Starting position: lie on your back, a small pillow under your head, but the back of your head slightly touches the floor, your arms are slightly moved away from your body, there is a bolster under your knees, your legs are slightly apart. You breathe freely and easily, while the lateral abdominal muscles are stretched.

2. Starting position: lying on back. You bend your legs at the knees, while your knees drop to the floor, first in one direction, then in the other. You inhale air through your nose and exhale through your mouth.

3. Starting position: lying on back. Feet rest on the floor. You transfer your body weight from the lower back to the tailbone and back.

4. Starting position: lie on your back, legs extended. One by one, lift your legs up, while rotating the ankle of the leg being lifted.

5. Starting position: stand on your knees, rest your palms on the floor, elbow joints are not bent. You arch your back, lowering your chin at the same time, and after a few seconds you straighten your back.

Remember: when doing physical exercise, you should not make sudden movements, you should not overtire yourself, and your breathing should always remain even.

10

Sexual relations during pregnancy

I t all depends on how you feel and the doctor's recommendations. If there are no medical contraindications, then you can not refuse sex until the 8th month of pregnancy.

However, if there is a threat of miscarriage, it is better not to have sex.

Most pregnant women experience a clear decrease in sexual desire, but in some cases, desire may remain the same or increase slightly.

Sexual intercourse during this period should not be frequent. Particular attention should be paid to your and your partner's personal hygiene, because an infection can get into the vagina. Sexual relations should be reduced to a minimum in the first three months of pregnancy, and excluded in the last two.

As for positions during sexual intercourse, a lateral position is recommended from the sixth month. The position in which the woman is on the bottom is not suitable during pregnancy.

Don't forget: the feeling that you are beautiful and loved creates the psychological comfort you need so much.

11

The importance of mental attitude

The nervous system is involved in all changes occurring in the body of the expectant mother. Brain activity is mobilized. A woman expecting a child reacts more sharply to external stimuli.

During pregnancy, you face a number of difficulties, which introduce anxiety and nervousness into your life.

The question that worries you most is: how will the birth go? Don't isolate yourself, an experienced obstetrician-gynecologist will dispel all your doubts.

Not the least place in your mind is occupied by thoughts about financial difficulties, housing problems, etc. Try to accurately assess the current situation. Remember that you have the right to special attention and support from loved ones, that you must take care of your peace of mind, avoid stress, and await the birth of your baby with joy, and not with fear.

12

Baby's arriving

Your baby might arrive earlier than expected, so it's worth having your hospital bag. It's never too early to start. Prepare a checklist, and print it out. Pack the bag with your partner, so you can double check the checklist and make sure you'll have everything you might need, and place them near the door, or in your car, so you'll be ready to go at a moment's notice.

Labor and delivery day checklist can be:

- Hospital paperwork, ID, and insurance card
- Key contact numbers and information
- Bathrobe
- Slippers and flip-flops.
- Hairbands or a headband/headscarf
- Socks
- Lip balm
- Body lotion or massage oil
- Water spray and sponge
- Comfortable pillow(s)

- Relaxing entertainment
- Eye mask and earplugs

Many of these things may help you relax a little bit, and be comfortable during labor and delivery, and it's a good idea to tower something loose and comfortable.

After delivery you will want to make yourself feel at home as much as possible.

The checklist after delivery bag can be:

- Underwear/big pants
- Heavy-duty maternity pads
- Nursing pads
- Nursing bra
- Open front pajamas
- Wheat bag
- Lavender oil
- Mints
- Birthing ball
- Nightgowns
- Washrag
- Toiletries
- Bras
- Glasses and skin care products
- Comfy Clothes
- Dark towels
- Handheld fan
- Cash
- Peri bottle
- Phone and charger

- Nipple creams
- Handouts and reference book
- Snacks and drinks

The hospital bag checklist for your baby:

- Bodysuit
- Diapers
- Socks and booties
- Receiving blanket
- Going-home outfit
- Car seat
- Baby wipes
- Sleepsuit
- Scratch mittens
- Booties or socks
- Newborn nappies x25
- Muslin squares x5
- Hat
- Baby snowsuit (if it is really cold outside)

If you're getting close to your due date, it's helpful to know how to time your contractions, if you lost your mucus plug, or break the water, as well as how to spot other signs of labor. Contact your healthcare provider if you think you're going into labor.

Congratulations! The birth of a new person is one of the most delightful mysteries of nature. You have a baby. Your baby has finally made his/her long-anticipated entrance into the big, wide world. How many questions arise: how to bathe, what to wear, when to feed, etc.

Being a mum to a newborn is probably the most mind-blowing thing you'll ever experience. But it is also the most brilliant journey. There are 12 baby care skills new parents need to know:

- Nappy changing
- Feeding
- Swaddling
- Topping and tailing
- Bonding
- Baby massage
- Soothing
- Using a sling or carrier
- Winding
- Bathing
- Holding
- Dressing

All your concerns can be resolved. Pay attention to the following tips and try to follow them.

When your baby is premature, to keep the baby warm, use a cotton sheet and cotton blanket, adding another blanket if the baby needs extra. Try to keep room temperature between 18-21 Celsius (64-69 Fahrenheit). Check the baby regularly to make sure she's not too hot or cold (by feeling the back of her neck or tummy). It's normal for a baby's hands and feet to feel colder than the rest of her body, though.

13

Children's "dowry"

By the time you return from the maternity hospital, the new family member should already have a so-called children's "dowry" ready, which you probably already bought or sewed yourself. Check everything carefully again. The children's dowry includes:

- 25 washcloth muslin cotton blankets, of which 15 are thin and 10 are flannelette. The size of the diaper is at least 120 x 120 cm (48 inches x 48 inches). The baby can get out of small blankets.
- 20 diapers. It is best to sew diapers from gauze fabric.
- 8 thin vests and 8 flannelettes. They are changed daily.
- 2 thin and 2 flannel caps. Put caps on your child when you go for a walk with him, and after giving him/her a bath. In the cold season, the cap is worn under a hat.
- 3 small scarves. The headscarf is worn, like a cap, under a cap.
- 2 blankets: 1 light and 1 warm.
- 1 large oilcloth and 2 small ones, size 30 x 30 cm (12 inches x 12 inches).

Wash all items in advance and iron them thoroughly. Blankets should be ironed through a piece of cotton or gauze cloth. It's highly recommended to use non-bio detergents for baby clothes (to avoid irritating your baby's sensitive skin). To prevent the fabric from becoming itchy for your little one's skin, a fabric softener can be a huge help.

14

Envelope or blanket

I f you doubt whether it is better for your baby to put him/her in an envelope when going for a walk, or to wrap them in a blanket, then know that both are acceptable.

It is important to wrap your baby correctly. Do not wrap it too tightly, especially in the chest area, as this may interfere with breathing.

Do not forget that movement contributes to the physical development of the baby.

15

Cleanliness is the key to health

Before you return with your newborn from the maternity hospital, the entire apartment must be cleaned with special care.

Particular attention should be paid to the children's room. There should be nothing superfluous in the room in which the child will live. It is better to remove flowers from the windowsill, as they interfere with the penetration of light. There should be no dust anywhere. Window glass should simply shine.

Wet cleaning in the children's room should be carried out daily. Of course, it is impossible to achieve complete sterility, but cleanliness is necessary.

Be sure to boil and iron the undershirts and diapers that come into contact with the not yet completely healed navel with a hot iron.

Boil all bottles, nipples, and pacifiers every morning. Boil them within 5 minutes. If the pacifier accidentally falls on the floor, it is enough to wash it with boiled water.

Remember one of the most important rules: never touch a child without washing your hands first. A young mother generally needs to wash her hands with soap as often as possible. Research has shown that the most common cause of children becoming infected with various infections, especially in the summer, is neglect of basic hygiene standards.

The baby needs fresh, cool air. Ventilate the room several times a day. Don't forget to cover the windows with gauze or nylon mesh to prevent the entry of mosquitoes, midges, and dust.

16

About bathing

From the moment the umbilical cord stump falls off until the child is 6 months old, it is necessary to bathe the baby every day, or a few times a week. At the same time, it is necessary to wash with soap no more than 2 times a week; on the other days, the baby is simply bathed in water.

Either boil water for bathing or add a solution of potassium permanganate to it; in this case, the water should be pale pink. Under no circumstances should powder crystals be thrown directly into a bathtub or basin, as they do not dissolve in water for a long time and can cause a burn on the child's skin. As for the bath itself, it, as well as the child's toys, must be washed with soap. But forget about the toys for now, the baby won't be interested in bath toys until they are a bit older.

The temperature of the water in which the child is bathed should be 36-38 degrees (96.8 - 100.4 degrees Fahrenheit). Please note that while you are undressing the child, the water will cool down by 1 degree (33.8 degrees Fahrenheit). After washing the child, rinse with water. The water temperature for rinsing is 35 degrees (95 degrees Fahrenheit).

The air temperature in the room during bathing should be 20-22 degrees (68 - 71.6 degrees Fahrenheit).

Starting from the second month after birth, the temperature of the water in the bath gradually increases to 34 degrees (93.2 degrees Fahrenheit).

A child who is six months old can be bathed every other day.

When bathing your baby, follow a certain sequence of actions.

1. Undress the child.

2. Lower the child into the water up to his shoulders. Water should not get into the ears, nose or mouth. Place the baby's head on your left forearm (if you are left-handed, then on your right) so that the back is on your palm.

3. With your free hand, pour over the baby's neck and chest for 2-3 minutes.

4. Lather your free hand with baby soap.

5. Carefully, without pressing, soap the child's head from the forehead to the back of the head.

6. Make sure that the soap does not get into the eyes.

7. Rinse the soap off the baby's head.

8. Using a very soft sponge, soaped with baby soap, wash the entire body.

9. Pay attention to the fact that behind the ears, under the arms, fingers, and groin must be washed very carefully.

10. Prepare boiled water in a separate container and wash the child's face with it.

11. Turn the baby onto his stomach and rinse the baby with clean water. Remember: when rinsing, water should be poured on the shoulders, not on the head.

12. Wrap your baby in a sheet. Wipe the baby with gentle movements. First of all, dry the head and hair using stroking movements, then the torso, and then between the legs.

Consider building your baby's bath time into the bedtime routine. It works perfectly, which will tell them that it's time to nod off. This won't work if the baby is tired or hungry though.

17

Oatmeal bath for your toddler and benefits

Your baby has very sensitive skin and natural products such as oatmeal have some amazing benefits for your baby's skin. An oat bath is a homemade, natural way of helping to aid, soothe different kinds of skin irritations, reducing redness. It is rich in calcium and vitamins that are great for your baby's skin. You can use many types of oats or plain oatmeal. Colloidal oatmeal is a perfect option. "Milk bath" is made from blended oatmeal of 100 g which looks like a fine powder and dissolved in hot-warm water. Oat bath can help soothe:

- Chickenpox
- Dry skin
- Hives
- Eczema
- Nappy rash

Let your baby soak in the bath for around 15-20 minutes to soothe those skin irritations. Your little one can have an oatmeal bath twice a day, as it will moisturize their dry skin.

18

Face needs to be washed

You need to wash your baby's face twice a day, morning and evening.

Sequence of actions when washing the face

1. Pour warm boiled water into a container, dip a piece of cotton wool or the tip of a soft towel into it.

2. Wipe the child's face, as well as the neck and behind the ears.

3. Prepare a solution of boric acid (1 teaspoon per glass of water).

4. Wash the eyes with cotton wool soaked in this solution, moving from the outer corner of the eye to the nose.

5. When rinsing the right eye, point the child's head to the right, and when rinsing the left eye, point it to the left to prevent water from penetrating from one eye to the other. It is important to remember that a separate piece of cotton wool is taken for each eye.

6. If you find whitish particles in the corners of your eyes, then you need to wash the eyes twice a day. In the morning and after the day.

7. Make flagella from cotton wool, moisten them with warm boiled water.

8. Insert the flagellum with careful screw-like movements into the

child's nostril. Use a separate piece of cotton wool for each nostril.

9. Clean the child's ears in the same way. Remember: to prevent damage to the thin, easily vulnerable skin of the ear canals, never use hard objects.

19

Trimming nails

Cutting the nails is a mandatory procedure that you should not be afraid of. For this, use separate small scissors with rounded edges, which should not be tight or loose. Before the procedure, scissors must be disinfected with alcohol or cologne.

There should be no hangnails on the child's fingers, as they can cause pustules to form.

Once every 7 days, for preventive purposes, lubricate the nail bed on the fingers and toes with a 2% alcohol solution of iodine.

20

How to avoid infection

At the beginning of life, staphylococcal and other infections pose a great danger to the child's health. Unfortunately, its source can sometimes be our maternity hospitals. But we should not forget about the dangers of postpartum pregnancy. Often a child becomes infected from the mother if she suffers from inflammatory diseases such as tonsillitis, pyelonephritis, cholecystitis and others.

The infection can enter the child's body during feeding. It is very important to monitor the condition of your mammary glands in order to prevent the occurrence of cracks in the nipples, the appearance and development of mastitis, since these things that bother you can serve as a source of infectious disease for your baby.

Infection with any infection can manifest itself in the formation of small pustular inflammations of the skin. Pustules usually appear on the head, under the armpits, in the groin area, and less often along the edge of the nail fold on the arms and legs. In this regard, every morning, after unwrapping the child, carefully examine him/her. The baby's skin should be smooth and light.

If you find any rashes on your baby's skin, contact the pediatrician immediately.

Please note that the reddish dotted rash is not dangerous - it is prickly heat, it means that you wrap your child too warmly at night.

A small vesicle with a whitish-yellow head is an abscess. If you see it in one place, it's too early to say it's an infection. Treat the abscess with a piece of cotton wool soaked in alcohol. Then burn it with brilliant green.

If you find several pustules at the same time, it is possible that an infection has entered the child's body.

The infection can also enter the baby's body through the umbilical wound. By the time of discharge from the maternity hospital, it should almost heal, only a dried crust remains. You need to keep this area clean and dry.

If the wound has not healed and ichor comes out of it, then it should be treated by a medical professional. Before the doctor arrives, you can drop a few drops of hydrogen peroxide into the wound, without touching it, and after foam appears on the wound, carefully dry it with sterile cotton wool and treat it with brilliant green.

21

Breastfeeding

I t is mother's milk that is the most complete form of nutrition for a child. The temperature of breast milk is the most suitable for the baby. Being in the mother's arms, feeling her smell and warmth, the child feels calm and protected, which improves the absorption of the food the baby receives. Breastfed babies should eat as much as they want, but a general rule of thumb is roughly 16 to 24 ounces of breast milk or formula in 24 hours.

It is in the process of feeding that the important beginnings of the emotional connection between the child and the mother are laid.

Breastfeeding rules.

1. Before you start feeding, the baby needs to be swaddled.

2. Wash your hands with soap.

3. Wash the nipple with warm boiled water.

4. Feed in a comfortable position. It is best to feed while sitting on a chair, leaning on the back.

5. When placing the baby on the left breast, place a stool under the left leg, and vice versa - under the right one if the baby is suckling on the right breast.

6. Make sure that the child grasps with his gums not only the tip of the nipple, but also the area around the nipple.

7. While holding your breasts from above and below, be careful, make sure that it does not fall on the baby's nose, interfering with oxygen access.

8. During one feeding, give the baby only one breast. This improves the process of milk formation. Start feeding both breasts at a time after 7-8 months, when the milk supply decreases.

9. It is advisable that a nursing mother's breasts be soft and pliable so that the baby gets full quickly.

10. If the child begins to suck too actively, then it is necessary to remove the nipple from time to time.

11. If the baby sucks too sluggishly, sleepily, then stroke their cheek, pull lightly on the nipple.

12. If, despite a sufficient amount of milk in the breast, the child sucks poorly and is clearly malnourished, pay attention to the nipple; most likely it is flat in shape. Try feeding your baby through the pad or stretch before each feeding nipple with fingers.

The reason for this child's behavior may be that your breasts are too tight.

In this case, express the first portions of milk, and then, when the breasts become more pliable, give it to the baby.

13. The baby may begin to suck greedily, but immediately releases the nipple, turns away, and screams.

Most often the reason is that he has a tummy ache.

A child experiences cramping pain in the abdomen most often during feeding, because the entry of food into the stomach reflexively causes defecation, accompanied by cramping contractions along the intestines.

Drink a glass of water to stay hydrated to ensure your body can make enough milk. Try to sleep when the baby sleeps. Eat regularly, because breastfeeding burns calories fast. Reduce stress. Stress produces a hormone called cortisol which reduces lactogenesis, and has a negative impact on your milk supply and let down.

Baby will lose weight after birth. Nearly all newborns will leave the hospital or birthing center weighing less than they first checked in.

22

Feeding time

Remember the most important thing - strictly adhere to feeding times. Milk is digested in the baby's stomach within three hours, the same time is necessary for the accumulation of new milk in the mother's breast. Your little one knows how much they need. Let your baby set the schedule. Breastfeeding works by supply and demand. BUT it is recommended to feed the baby every 3 hours until 3 months of age, from 3 to 6 months - every three and a half hours, after 6 months - every 4 hours. Anticipate your baby's needs. Rather than waiting for your baby to cry, try and look for other signs that they're hungry, like raising their head a lot or opening and closing their mouth.

At night you should take a long break of at least 6 hours.

Babies quickly adapt to the routine to which they are accustomed. Therefore, from the very beginning it is necessary to adhere to a certain routine and not deviate from it.

If you are unable to breastfeed your baby at the right time, you need to express milk for this feeding using a breast pump. Consult your doctor about this.

Expressed milk should be labeled, dated and stored in a completely clean bottle or in breast milk storage bags in a cool place like refrigerator

(up to 5 days at 4 celsius or lower), in the ice compartment of the fridge (for two weeks) or in the freezer (you can freeze it up to six months, but use it within 24 hours after defrosting). To defrost the breast milk, you have to do it slowly in the fridge which could take up to 12 hours, or popping it in a jug of warm water or holding it under warm running water, then shaking it well, use it straight away. Do not re-freeze milk that has been defrosted. Benefits of storing breast milk can be:

- So your partner can help with feeding
- If you're unable to breastfeed because you're at work or otherwise engaged.
- To relieve the pressure of sore breasts and nipples
- If you're power pumping to boost your milk supply
- If your baby is struggling with latching but you would like to feed your baby with your breast milk.

Before feeding, warm it up a little by dipping the bottle in warm water.

Do not let the milk stagnate; After each feeding, express it to the last drop. Make sure that the child does not crush the nipple in the mouth or suck on the side.

Breastfeed your baby for 20-25 minutes.

At the end of feeding, do not suddenly remove the nipple from the baby's mouth, but press lightly on the baby's chin or pinch the nose for a second.

After feeding, lubricate the nipples with vitamin A, and at night with any vegetable oil, preheating it in a water bath.

Take air baths, they are very beneficial for the chest (several times a day for 20-30 minutes).

It is normal for nipples to be sore about three to seven days into breastfeeding. If your baby is in the correct position and latched properly, breastfeeding shouldn't be all that pain. If you've just started breastfeeding, keep an eye on your nipples after the first few feeds - they will be a good indicator as to whether or not everything is ok . If it is still not possible to avoid cracks in the nipples, you need to reduce the load on the nipples, express milk more often, and feed the baby from a bottle. You can also use a special breastfeeding pad. The ways to soothe sore nipples. **A few recommendations for the prevention of cracked nipples and the development of mastitis.**

- Get the right position
- Reduce engorgement
- Relax your nipples (apply a hot wet cloth)
- Change the bra
- Apply your own milk
- Avoid using soap
- Go topless
- Choose the right breast pads
- Go natural

1. Manuka honey (but wash the nipples well before feeding baby)
2. Olive oil
3. Use silver nipple cups

- Check your breast pump shield

23

About mixed and artificial feeding

If you don't have enough or no milk at all, then you need to switch to mixed or artificial feeding. Currently, there are special milk formulas for babies under one year old, the composition of which is as close as possible to breast milk. These mixtures, which have a complex composition, not only contain proteins, fats, and carbohydrates in the required ratio, but are also enriched with minerals and vitamins.

Of course, artificial nutrition is not an equivalent replacement, but if you have to choose, choose the best. In the first months of life, feed your baby one of these adapted formulas that you have chosen. Select the desired mixture experimentally. The baby eats suitable food with appetite, while gaining weight, and the baby's stool remains normal.

Do not buy several different types of baby food at the same time. To begin with, choose one, and if it suits the baby, stock up on some of it. If not, try another one.

Remember that frequent changes of infant formula can cause intestinal disorders.

With mixed feeding, supplementary feeding is given after breastfeeding so that the baby sucks the maximum amount of mother's milk.

24

Feeding the baby

It is necessary to feed a baby from the fourth month of life, since the baby is no longer getting enough of the substances contained in mother's milk or artificial milk formula.

The time has come to add ordinary human food to their diet: vegetable puree, porridge, cottage cheese, and later meat broth, meat, bread. This is complementary feeding.

During complementary feeding, the baby switches from liquid food to semi-liquid and then thick food. In this regard, the work of the digestive system is activated.

To begin with, give your baby a minimum amount of porridge, blended meat and vegetable puree. You need to start with one or two teaspoons, gradually increasing the portion over 10-12 days.

Remember that you should never give more than one new dish in one day.

Give complementary foods before breastfeeding, as a child who is hungry will be more willing to eat food that is new to them. Give your child complementary foods in the first year of life, guided by various schemes that present the sequence of introducing new foods into the child's diet, their volume and periodicity of feedings.

Keep in mind that the total amount of food included in a child's diet in the second half of their life becomes practically unchanged and amounts to no more than 1000 grams per day.

At the first and last feeding, the child should be given only light food throughout the year: mother's milk or artificial milk formula, and after 10 months - kefir, whole milk.

From the age of 11 months, at 8 pm a child can be offered vegetable puree or porridge as a main course, and the baby only drinks it down with kefir or a formula.

Night feeding at 10 pm is not mandatory; if the baby is against it, then you don't have to insist.

25

Baby probiotics

P robiotics are often described as "good bacteria" when given in the right amount, which can have health benefits. Probiotics are generally considered to be safe for healthy individuals, including babies. Conditions for the use of probiotics:

- If the baby has colic
- If you want to help prevent or minimize antibiotic-associated diarrhea
- If your baby has acute gastroenteritis
- The babies who experience constipation and abdominal pain

There are typically minimal or no side effects experienced from probiotics. A small number of babies or children may experience a short-term change in their bowel habits. Always choose to discuss with the professional Doctor.

26

Cradle cap

If your baby has a skin condition of patches of white or yellow scales on their head, they might have a cradle cap. There are plenty of simple ways to help to clear it up. It is also known as infantile seborrheic dermatitis. The skin can also look greasy, flaky and occasionally red. 50% of babies under eight months old will go away on their own within six to 12 months. But if you want to help to get rid of it, there are several methods that you can try to ease cradle cap symptoms.

- Gentle rubbing with baby oil into your baby's scalp and leave overnight. In the morning use a soft baby brush to gently massage the area and wash it off
- It can help loosen scaly patches on the baby's head by using special cradle cap shampoo

27

Baby massage benefits

Baby massage is proven to be hugely beneficial for your baby's early development, as it promotes bilateral movements for your baby which means your baby is using both sides of the body and brain. After the massage they sleep longer and deeper, stress behaviors are reduced, motor development is improved, bonding process starts between mom and baby, it encourages eye to eye contact, smiling and mutual interaction which is a great way to bond with your baby, and can also help babies who suffer from sleep problems to relax and it reduces crying and irritability. Including some simple baby massage techniques into your baby's daily bedtime and bathing routine could help relieve some of the discomfort caused by colic.

Clean your hands before applying the oil. Apply the oil to your hands and rub hands together to warm it up before touching the baby's skin.

There are times when it is not advised to massage a baby.

1. Feeling unwell/having an off day
2. Has a fever
3. Has many skin conditions, lumps, bumps or rashes
4. No tummy massage directly after a feed/better to wait 40 minutes

5. Has any undiagnosed illness
6. If your baby is under a medical team

28

Ear cleaning

As the ears are a delicate part of the body, you may be unsure how to clean them and whether or not you even should clean them. Some babies will produce more earwax than others and it can vary in color from yellow to brown, and also varies in texture. It can be sticky and moist or dry and flaky. They will come out on their own. If you see some on the outer ear you can wipe it when cleaning with the baby bath towel or cotton wool, but avoid putting anything into the ear and don't use any ear wax remedies.

Start by dampening a cotton wool ball or pad or a soft flannel with clean warm water without soap. Wipe behind and around your baby's ear gently, then pat their ears dry with a clean towel.

29

Baby's head is flat

A baby's head grows very quickly in the first 4 months to accommodate the rapidly-growing brain. Small babies spend a lot of time sleeping - as much as 12 hours during the night (intervally waking up to be fed). When a baby lies continually on the same side of the head, growth is discouraged at that spot and redirected to the side on which the baby does not lie, creating asymmetry. In a baby who doesn't not move their head to either side, flattening will develop at the back of the head.

Flat patch on your baby's head is really manageable and treats itself. Completely natural condition that affects many babies, and is nothing to worry about. It has increased since doctors placed an emphasis on putting babies on their backs to sleep in order to reduce the risk of SIDS (Sudden Infant Death Syndrome). A young baby's skull is really soft and pliable, which means that it can get molded into a slightly different shape if there is constant pressure on part of the head. Since your baby spends most of the time lying down on their back, their head may naturally become flattened on the part that is bearing most of their weight. Your baby's head will naturally start to round off as they grow and start to move around but there are a few things you can do to help this process.

1. Put your baby's head in different positions to take pressure off the affected area.
2. Encourage them to look around as much as possible by moving toys.
3. Try to alternate the side you hold your baby when carrying and feeding them.
4. Sitting them up in things like a baby bean bag can also help, as the beans mold around your baby's head.
5. One of the options can be repositioning which is unpredictable and largely ineffective.
6. The other solution is to alter the surface on which the baby rests. There are many pillows sold for this purpose.
7. Encourage some tummy time every day (start with short sessions and build the length of time up to at least 20 minutes) by the time the baby is between three and four months old.

By the time they are one or two years old, any flattening will be hardly noticeable. There are no long-term side effects for babies with flat head syndrome and your baby will not experience any pain or other symptoms either.

30

Bonding with your baby

The moment you first bond with your baby is unforgettable - whether it is during pregnancy, the first time you lay eyes on them, or months later when you've got to know each other. Bonding is the emotional connection you have with your baby. Babies need loving relationships to properly develop emotionally and physically. Try not to worry if you haven't bonded with your baby yet. The average time it takes parents to establish a connection is six and a half months. Consistency of care is important for mother-baby bonding. After being a parent, there are plenty of ways to bond with your baby.

- Skin-to-skin contact

Most moms love cuddling their little one or holding them close. Skin-to-skin contact is a great way to bond with your newborn. After the birth, the baby is placed directly on the mother's chest. Holding your baby close to your skin helps boost your baby's immune system, it keeps their energy levels stable, it keeps them calm, it encourages your baby's brain to develop, regulates their body temperature, and promotes breastfeeding.

- Breastfeeding

It can be a wonderfully fulfilling, bonding experience and is the start of your incredible journey getting to know your baby.

- Eye contact

Babies are drawn to faces. Maintain eye contact while feeding, talking, or playing with your baby. This helps them feel secure, protected, and connected.

- Respond and react to cues

Be careful to pay attention to your baby's cues and respond quickly. It can be hunger, tiredness, and a need for a nappy change. It builds trust and security.

- Talk to your baby

Your baby will respond to the rhythm and tone of your voice. Sing songs, or just talk to your baby. This will turn to your favorite activity to do with your little one.

- Hold and cuddle

Hold them, cuddle them, let them feel warmth and comfort of your embrace. Physical touch is a powerful way to bond with your baby.

- Establish routines

Daily routines can help your baby feel secure and create special moments for bonding, such as bedtime rituals.

- Baby massage

Massaging your baby can be a soothing and bonding experience. Use gentle, slow strokes, and ensure the room is comfortable and warm.

- Include other family members

This not only strengthens the overall family bond but also provides a support system for both you and the baby.

- Playtime

Playing with soft toys, making funny faces, or even playing peek-a-boo fosters a sense of joy and connection.

- Be patient and flexible

Building a strong bond takes time. Be patient and flexible, adjusting to your baby's needs and cues. Each baby is unique, so what works for one may not work for another.

31

My baby is crying

Along with your instincts as a mom - no one knows your baby quite well as you. Here are the main crying cues:

1. Hunger (The baby may suck her fist or fingers, stick their tongue out, smack her lips)
2. Discomfort (The baby may be restless and unsettled)
3. Tiredness (The baby may be restless and rub her eyes, which may look glazed)
4. Pain (The baby's cry may be harsh, high-pitched and intense from the start)
5. Fear (The baby's eyes may stay mostly open she cries)
6. Too much stimulation (Jerky movements may be noticeable and she might turn her head away from you or try to bat things away with her hands)
7. Wind or colic (She may fidget, squirm, grimace and draw her knees to her chest)
8. Feeling sick (Most moms will recognise this cry as not quite right or different from normal)
9. Time to change diaper

10. Wants a cuddle
11. The baby is too hot

One of the crying is Controlled Crying - This helps your baby settle themselves, or learn to self soothe. It is a way to teach a baby to fall asleep on their own after crying for a few minutes. It means that they will not rely on you to soothe them whenever they wake up. You need to wait until your baby is six months old to try this out.

32

Baby starts teething

All babies start teething at different ages of months and teething can last for different periods of time. You may start to notice the symptoms, their first tooth can take until 6 months old, and teething lasts until they are about 25-33 months. It will take around 8 days for the tooth to push through the top layer of the gym (which can cause some discomfort) and a few months to continue to grow till the full size. When a tooth is ready to come through the gum, you'll be able to see its white tip just underneath the gum line. It is useful to know what signs to look out for when the baby starts teething.

Teething symptoms:

- Ear rubbing
- Biting
- Dribbles
- Irritability
- Chewing
- 1 flushed cheek
- A mild temperature of 38C
- Excess saliva production

- Not sleeping well
- Rubbing cheeks
- Nappy rash
- Refusing to eat
- Red and sore looking gum

It can be painful for babies. With some teeth, your baby might not feel up to feeding, as the suction can make their sore gums feel worse. They might also refuse solid food. Some teeth might cause a run of restless nights. Your baby may also bite to relieve the pressure in their gums. There are some ways that will ease the discomfort. Teething remedies can help your baby when they need it, from teething rings to gels. Experiment with teething toys is just the right pressure to ease the discomfort. A teething necklace can also be a great option for on the go. Paracetamol is best for relieving mild to moderate discomfort before a tooth comes through. When the baby is actually cutting a tooth, ibuprofen is more effective as it helps reduce the inflammation. Just recommend dosage and check with your doctor. Teething granules are a natural pain reliever to ease the pain and easily dissolve in the baby's mouth.

To numb your baby's gums, give them a teether that's been chilled in the fridge for half an hour. Give your baby a clean flannel soaked in warm water to suck on. Depending on the baby's age, feed chilled fruit purees or pop a chunk of frozen banana or plums in a baby feeder mesh bag. Wash your hands and crook of your little finger that will make a great teether, or gently press on her gum with your little finger.

You can start brushing your baby's teeth as soon as they start to come through.

33

Baby's speech and communication

Crying is your baby's first kind of communication they can do. In the first month or two, you will notice them making little sounds. Most babies can be taught how to use their hands to communicate before they can learn how to start talking as they naturally like to copy actions and movements from the people around them. But the main communication that they will start with crying, then the "oohing" and "ahhing" then they will recognise words and the sounds of your voice which will result in them "babbling" which could be "mama" or "dada". Around 6 months old is the most common time for this first word, but it can happen sooner or later than this. After that they will begin to pick up more words from you and everyone else around you. Babies love to listen to your voice, so talk, sing and coo, make eye contact as you go. Hold your baby close, look at them and chat about what you are doing. Repeat the sounds your baby makes back to them.

34

Baby's acting phases

Tummy time

It is where you lay your baby on their stomach for brief periods while they are awake to help strengthen their neck and shoulder muscles and improve their motor skills in preparation for crawling and when the baby starts rolling over.

Tummy time is a brilliant way of helping your baby to gain strength to build all the important muscles they need for sitting, crawling, it develops muscle strength, encourages head control, helps to prevent baby flat head, eases gas pain, stimulates senses and cognitive development, helps hand eye coordination and visual development, develops motor skills, helps baby and parents bond, establishes a routine. They will not have fun being on tummy time until the muscles in their neck are better developed. Once a baby can lift their head, they'll begin to really enjoy the freedom and love the view.

Baby's head is up

It is important to keep the baby's head supported. During those first few months when the baby doesn't have control of their neck muscles, it can be a rather anxious time. But it will not be long until the baby is comfortable and confidently supports their own head. At around three months old, your baby will have developed enough strength in their neck to keep their heads partially upright. Between 3-6 months muscles will only strengthen, and by six months, they should be able to fully control their neck muscles and have fully head control. Tummy time is a great activity to help build those neck muscles from a young age. Some babies begin tummy time from one month old. Tummy time is a great opportunity to notice your baby trying to turn their head, too.

The next step is lifting both the head and chest. This usually happens in month one to three. The more they get used to tummy time, the more likely they are to begin to push themselves up with their elbows and arms (the first step to crawling).

Baby starts rolling over

Generally, babies start the journey by rocking on their stomachs at around 5 months old.This is them starting to practice those all-important muscle movements that are required to roll over. Between 6-8 months, the baby will give rolling over a try. Most start by rolling from their tummy into their back. They quickly learn to roll over from front to back too. By eight months, your baby will most likely be rolling over easily. There is nothing wrong with giving your baby some help with rolling over.

Baby sits up

Most of the time, babies sit up on their own. Typically, they learn to sit up between 4 and 8 months old. Your baby has already mastered rolling over and holding their heads up at this stage. So you can expect them to sit up for a couple of minutes without support, by the time they're 8 months old.

Baby starts crawling

The first few months of babyhood go by so quickly, and before you know it, you can see those little legs getting eager to move. Most babies start to crawl between 7 months to 10 months old after they've learnt to sit up, or they might skip the phase entirely and start pulling themselves up to learn how to walk. Help your baby to crawl:

- Give them plenty of tummy time
- Make sure there's plenty of space
- Encourage them to reach for toys
- Help them to move

Each baby has a different way of crawling style: from the crab crawl to the bottom scoot crawl. Some babies crawl backwards before they crawl forwards. Once your baby is on the move, you'll need to ensure their new world is ready to explore safely. As with everything, you'll need to keep a close eye on your little adventurer at all times, because they will not sit still in one place!

Don't push your baby to crawling. They aren't ready as it can slow down the development. Just gentle encouragement will just help them figure it out.

Baby starts walking

The moment your baby gets up on two legs and walks one step, two steps - on their own represents the culmination of months of hard work that displayed coordination, balance, and bravery. This will help them be able to sit up, with a little help from you before they can do it alone. This tends to take place between four and seven months. While you will be able to gently pull your child up to help them stand after they've nailed sitting up, they most likely won't be able to do it on their own until between nine months and a year. It can start from them pulling themselves up from anything they can grip such as the sofa or even your legs. At this point, they will probably only be able to stand briefly before falling and landing backwards onto their bum.

Some babies start to walk as early as nine months old, most tend to start at about one year and some babies don't feel the need to get up until they're 18 months old. Babies are individuals. Do not push them to go too far, too fast. And when they start walking, let them do as much as they can on their own, at their own speed. They need to do it to learn about coordination, balance, and what their body can do. Soft surface to walk on, shoe-free time, holding them at the hips can help the baby walk.

Stages of learning to walk

- Step one - Head control (Between 3-6 weeks old)
- Step two - Body awareness (Between 2-5 months old0
- Step three - Rolling (Between 3-6 months old)
- Step four - Sitting (Between 6-8 months old)
- Step five - The four-point pose
- Step six - Crawling (Between 6-12 months old)
- Step seven - High kneel and cruising
- Step eight - Walking!

35

Baby starts sleeping on their stomach

As a parent, you're probably constantly worried about the baby rolling onto their belly while they sleep. Is putting the baby to sleep on their back really best, or can they sleep on their tummy? It is not okay for babies to sleep on their stomach. It means they will breathe in less air, which can increase their chance of Sudden Infant Death Syndrome (SIDS). The best and only position for a baby to sleep is on their back. If they sleep on their side, they can easily roll onto their stomach. Once they are able to roll themselves over, it is safe for them to sleep on their stomach. Not all babies wait until the six months mark to roll over, but some as young as 3 or 4 months can turn onto their stomach while they're sleeping. Just gently turn the baby onto their back. But it is recommended to put the babies to sleep on their back until their first birthdays.

36

Grandma's legacy/Nursery Rhymes

Little babies react sensitively to their mother's voice.

Even the most turbulent baby will quickly calm down when they hear the calm voice of the person closest to them.

Therefore, try to talk with your baby more often from the first days of their life. Kind and gentle words will help your baby grow up responsive and sensitive. And nursery rhymes and songs, familiar to our grandmothers, will be your baby's first acquaintance with beautiful and diverse literature.

Turn reading these short poems into a game, activities with nursery rhymes can turn reading into a learning playtime event, making the rhyme fun with clapping to the rhythm of the verse, finger paints, creating great artwork, dance, noise or play acting out the characters makes learning the rhyme a delightful experience, and in a fairly short time your baby will easily repeat familiar lines after you. Kids love to play as they learn. As they grow, try different ideas along with rhymes to bring out their creativity and stretch their imaginations. The creativity, hand & finger play activities for nursery rhymes not only make the rhyme more fun, but will bring more benefits with lots of development for your special little one. The more interesting and fun learning can be, the more likely your little one will enjoy the learning.

Today, nursery rhymes can be shared with our children and grandchildren through books, songs, activities, parties, gifts and decor!

Pat a Cake

Pat-a-cake, pat-a-cake baker's man
Bake me a cake as fast as you can
Pat it and prick it and mark it with "B"
Put it in the oven for baby and me
For baby and me
For baby and me
And there will be plenty for baby and me
Pat-a-cake, pat-a-cake baker's man
Bake me a cake as fast as you can
Pat it and prick it and mark it with "B"
Put it in the oven for baby and me
For baby and me
For baby and me
And there will be plenty for baby and me

The Itsy Bitsy Spider

The itsy bitsy spider crawled up the water spout.
Down came the rain, and washed the spider out.
Out came the sun, and dried up all the rain,
and the itsy bitsy spider went up the spout again.

Twinkle

Twinkle, twinkle, little star,

How I wonder what you are!
Up above the world so high,
Like a diamond in the sky.

When the blazing sun is gone,
When he nothing shines upon,
Then you show your little light,
Twinkle, twinkle, all the night.

Then the traveler in the dark,
Thanks you for your tiny spark,
He could not see which way to go,
If you did not twinkle so.

In the dark blue sky you keep,
And often thro' my curtains peep,
For you never shut your eye,
Till the sun is in the sky.

'Tis your bright and tiny spark,
Lights the traveler in the dark:
Tho' I know not what you are,
Twinkle, twinkle, little star.

All the leaves are falling down
All the leaves are falling down,
Orange, yellow, red and brown,
Falling softly as they do,
Over me and over you,
All the leaves are falling down,

Orange, yellow, red and brown.

Snowflake

Snowflake, snowflake, little snowflake.
Little snowflake falling from the sky.
Snowflake, snowflake, little snowflake.
Falling, falling, falling, falling, falling,
falling, falling, falling, falling…
falling on my head.
Snowflake, snowflake, little snowflake.
Little snowflake falling from the sky.
Snowflake, snowflake, little snowflake.
Falling, falling, falling, falling, falling,
falling, falling, falling, falling…
falling on my nose.
Snowflake, snowflake, little snowflake.
Little snowflake falling from the sky.
Snowflake, snowflake, little snowflake.
Falling, falling, falling, falling, falling,
falling, falling, falling, falling…
falling in my hand.
Falling on my head.
Falling on my nose.
Falling in my hand.
Snowflake, snowflake, little snowflake…

Old MacDonald

Old MacDonald had a farm
Ee i ee i o

And on his farm he had some cows
Ee i ee i oh
With a moo-moo here
And a moo-moo there
Here a moo, there a moo
Everywhere a moo-moo
Old MacDonald had a farm
Ee i ee i o
Old MacDonald had a farm
Ee i ee i o
And on his farm he had some chicks
Ee i ee i o
With a cluck-cluck here
And a cluck-cluck there
Here a cluck, there a cluck
Everywhere a cluck-cluck
Old MacDonald had a farm
Ee i ee i o
Old MacDonald had a farm
Ee i ee i o
And on his farm he had some pigs
Ee i ee i o
With an oink-oink here
And an oink-oink there
Here an oink, there an oink
Everywhere an oink-oink
Old MacDonald had a farm
Ee i ee i o

Buttons

Buttons! Buttons, a farthing a pair,
Come, who will buy them of me?
They're round and sound and pretty,
And fit for the girls of the city.
Come, who will buy them of me?
Buttons! Buttons, a farthing a pair.

37

Lullabies

Sleep is important for any person. And for a child, good sleep is even more important. A sleep-deprived baby causes problems for parents. And they don't feel very good either. Therefore, put your child to bed at the appropriate time. It is not always easy to carry out this good intention. But if the child is accustomed to going to bed at the same time, then they will already be partially prepared for sleep. Never force someone to sleep. Patiently but persistently persuade your child to finish the game and go to bed. There's no sweeter way to put your baby to bed than with a soothing lullaby. Read them a story or sing a lullaby before bed. Singing lullabies or songs to your baby is a lovely, sweet way to soothe them down, that will calm the child and set them up for sleep when bedtime approaches. It can be a key part of your little one's bedtime routine, letting them know that the bed time for sleep is coming soon. Newborns up to 3 or 4 months old need 14 to 17 hours of sleep in a 24-hour period, usually waking up every two to four hours to eat. Whenever possible, sing a lullaby to your baby yourself, rather than playing it on a device. Parents' voices (especially mothers' voices) engage babies' brains far better than other sounds. The child will fall asleep calmly, and nothing will prevent them from seeing beautiful dreams and having a good rest. Never put headphones on your infant. If using a device to play lullabies for your baby, be sure to keep the volume low. Your child's inner ears are very sensitive, and anything above 85 decibels can cause hearing loss. Keep in mind that normal conversation is around 60 decibels.

"Rock-a-Bye Baby"
>Rock a bye baby, on the tree top,
>When the wind blows the cradle will rock.
>When the bough breaks the cradle will fall,
>And down will come baby, cradle and all.

Rock a bye baby, gently you swing,
>Over the cradle, Mother will sing,
>Sweet is the lullaby over your nest
>That tenderly sings my baby to rest.

From the high rooftops, down to the sea
>No one's as dear as baby to me
>Wee little hands, eyes shiny and bright
>Now sound asleep until morning light

Rock a bye baby, on the tree top,
>When the wind blows the cradle will rock.
>When the bough breaks the cradle will fall,
>And down will come baby, cradle and all.

"Good Night"
>Now it's time to say good night,

Good night, sleep tight.
Now the sun turns out his light,
Good night, sleep tight.
Dream sweet dreams for me,
Dream sweet dreams for you.
Close your eyes and I'll close mine,
Good night, sleep tight.
Now the moon begins to shine,
Good night, sleep tight.
Dream sweet dreams for me,
Dream sweet dreams for you.
Close your eyes and I'll close mine,
Good night, sleep tight.
Now the sun turns out his light,
Good night, sleep tight.
Dream sweet dreams for me,
Dream sweet dreams for you.
Good night,
Good night, everybody,
Everybody, everywhere,
Good night.

"Cradle Song" ("Brahms' Lullaby")
Lullaby and good night,
With roses bestride.
Creep into thy bed,
There pillow thy head.
If God will thou shalt wake,
When the morning doth break.
If God will thou shalt wake,

When the morning doth break.
Lullaby and good night,
Those blue eyes close tight.
Bright angels are near,
So sleep without fear.
They will guard thee from harm,
With fair dreamland's sweet charm.
They will guard thee from harm,
With fair dreamland's sweet charm.

"Amazing Grace"
Amazing grace, how sweet the sound
That saved a wretch like me
I once was lost, but now am found
Was blind, but now I see
Was grace that taught my heart to fear
And grace, my fears relieved
How precious did that grace appear
The hour I first believed
Through many dangers, toils and snares
We have already come
T'was grace that brought us safe thus far
And grace will lead us home
And grace will lead us home
Amazing grace, how sweet the sound
That saved a wretch like me
I once was lost, but now am found
Was blind, but now I see
Was blind, but now I see

"Goodnight Sweetheart Goodnight"

Goodnight, sweetheart, well it's time to go,
Goodnight, sweetheart, well it's time to go,
I hate to leave you, but I really must say,
Goodnight, sweetheart, goodnight.
Goodnight, sweetheart, well it's time to go,
Goodnight, sweetheart, well it's time to go,
I hate to leave you, but I really must say,
Goodnight, sweetheart, goodnight.
Well, it's three o'clock in the morning,
Baby, I just can't treat you right.
Well, I hate to leave you, baby,
Don't mean maybe, because I love you so.
Goodnight, sweetheart, well it's time to go,
I hate to leave you, but I really must say,
Goodnight, sweetheart, goodnight.
Goodnight, sweetheart, well it's time to go,
Goodnight, sweetheart, well it's time to go,
I hate to leave you, but I really must say,
Goodnight, sweetheart, goodnight.
Now, my mother and my father,
Might hear if I stay here too long.
One kiss and we'll part,
And you'll be going,
You know I hate to see you go.

"Frère Jacque"

Frère Jacques, Frère Jacques,
Dormez-vous? Dormez-vous?
Sonnez les matines! Sonnez les matines!

Ding, dang, dong. Ding, dang, dong.

"Brother John"
Are you sleeping? Are you sleeping?
Brother John, Brother John,
Morning bells are ringing! Morning bells are ringing!
Ding, dang, dong. Ding, dang, dong.

"Swing Low, Sweet Chariot"
Swing low, sweet chariot
Coming for to carry me home
Swing low, sweet chariot
Coming for to carry me home
I looked over Jordan and what did I see
Coming for to carry me home
A band of angels coming after me
Coming for to carry me home
Swing low, sweet chariot
Coming for to carry me home
Swing low, sweet chariot
Coming for to carry me home
If you get there before I do
Coming for to carry me home
Tell all my friends I'm coming too
Coming for to carry me home
Swing low, sweet chariot
Coming for to carry me home
Swing low, sweet chariot
Coming for to carry me home

"Star Light, Star Bright"
Star light, star bright,
The first star I see tonight;
I wish I may, I wish I might,
Have the wish I wish tonight.

"Somewhere Over the Rainbow"
Somewhere over the rainbow
Way up high
There's a land that I heard of
Once in a lullaby
Somewhere over the rainbow
Skies are blue
And the dreams that you dare to dream
Really do come true
Someday I'll wish upon a star
And wake up where the clouds are far
Behind me
Where troubles melt like lemon drops
Away above the chimney tops
That's where you'll find me
Somewhere over the rainbow
Bluebirds fly
Birds fly over the rainbow
Why then, oh why can't I?
If happy little bluebirds fly
Beyond the rainbow
Why, oh why can't I?

"Lullaby (Goodnight, My Angel)"
  Goodnight, my angel, time to close your eyes,
  And save these questions for another day.
  I think I know what you've been asking me,
  I think you know what I've been trying to say.
  I promised I would never leave you,
  Then you should always know,
  Wherever you may go, no matter where you are,
  I never will be far away.
  Goodnight, my angel, now it's time to sleep,
  And still so many things I want to say.
  Remember all the songs you sang for me,
  When we went sailing on an emerald bay.
  And like a boat out on the ocean,
  I'm rocking you to sleep.
  The water's dark and deep, inside this ancient heart,
  You'll always be a part of me.
  Goodnight, my angel, now it's time to dream,
  And dream how wonderful your life will be.
  Someday your child may cry, and if you sing this lullaby,
  Then in your heart there will always be a part of me.
  Someday we'll all be gone,
  But lullabies go on and on,
  They never die,
  That's how you and I will be.

"All the Pretty Horses"
  Hush-a-bye, don't you cry.
  Go to sleepy little baby.
  When you wake, you shall have

All the pretty little horses.
Black and bays, dapples and grays,
Coach and six-a-little horses.
Hush-a-bye, don't you cry.
Go to sleepy little baby.
Hush-a-bye, don't you cry.
Go to sleepy little baby.
When you wake you shall have,
All the pretty little horses.
Black and bays, dapples and grays,
Coach and six-a-little horses.
Hush-a-bye, don't you cry.
Go to sleepy little baby.

"You Are My Sunshine"
You are my sunshine, my only sunshine,
You make me happy when skies are grey.
You'll never know, dear, how much I love you,
Please don't take my sunshine away.
The other night, dear, as I lay sleeping,
I dreamt I held you in my arms.
When I awoke, dear, I was mistaken,
So I hung my head, and I cried.
You are my sunshine, my only sunshine,
You make me happy when skies are grey.
You'll never know, dear, how much I love you,
Please don't take my sunshine away.
I'll always love you and make you happy,
If you will only say the same.
But if you leave me to love another,

You'll regret it all one day.
You are my sunshine, my only sunshine,
You make me happy when skies are grey.
You'll never know, dear, how much I love you,
Please don't take my sunshine away.
Please don't take my sunshine away.

"Hush, Little Baby"
Hush, little baby, don't say a word,
Papa's gonna buy you a mockingbird.
And if that mockingbird won't sing,
Papa's gonna buy you a diamond ring.
And if that diamond ring turns to brass,
Papa's gonna buy you a looking glass.
And if that looking glass gets broke,
Papa's gonna buy you a billy goat.
And if that billy goat won't pull,
Papa's gonna buy you a cart and bull.
And if that cart and bull turn over,
Papa's gonna buy you a dog named Rover.
And if that dog named Rover won't bark,
Papa's gonna buy you a horse and cart.
And if that horse and cart fall down,
You'll still be the sweetest little baby in town!

"Row, Row, Row Your Boat"
Row, row, row your boat
Gently down the stream
Merrily, merrily, merrily, merrily

Life is but a dream
(repeat four times)

"A Dream Is a Wish Your Heart Makes"

A dream is a wish your heart makes
When you're fast asleep
In dreams you will lose your heartaches
Whatever you wish for, you keep
Have faith in your dreams, and someday
Your rainbow will come smiling through
No matter how your heart is grieving
If you keep on believing
The dream that you wish will come true
A dream is a wish your heart makes
When you're fast asleep
In dreams you will lose your heartaches
Whatever you wish for, you keep
Have faith in your dreams, and someday
Your rainbow will come smiling through
No matter how your heart is grieving
If you keep on believing
The dream that you wish will come true

"Isn't She Lovely"

Isn't she lovely?
Isn't she wonderful?
Isn't she precious?
Less than one minute old
I never thought through love we'd be

Making one as lovely as she
But isn't she lovely made from love?
Isn't she pretty?
Truly the angel's best
Boy, I'm so happy
We have been heaven-blessed
I can't believe what God has done
Through us He's given life to one
But isn't she lovely made from love?
Isn't she lovely?
Life and love are the same
Life is Aisha,
The meaning of her name
Londie, it could have not been done
Without you who conceived the one
That's so very lovely, made from love, hey!

"Beautiful Boy (Darling Boy)"
Close your eyes
Have no fear
The monster's gone
He's on the run and your daddy's here
Beautiful, beautiful, beautiful
Beautiful boy
Beautiful, beautiful, beautiful
Beautiful boy
Before you go to sleep
Say a little prayer
Every day in every way, it's getting better and better
Beautiful, beautiful, beautiful

Beautiful boy
Beautiful, beautiful, beautiful
Beautiful boy
Out on the ocean sailing away
I can hardly wait
To see you come of age
But I guess we'll both just have to be patient
'Cause it's a long way to go
A hard row to hoe
Yes, it's a long way to go
But in the meantime
Before you cross the street
Take my hand
Life is what happens to you while you're busy making other plans
Beautiful, beautiful, beautiful
Beautiful boy
Beautiful, beautiful, beautiful
Beautiful boy
Before you go to sleep
Say a little prayer
Every day in every way, it's getting better and better
Beautiful, beautiful, beautiful
Beautiful boy
Darling, darling, darling
Darling Sean

"Didn't Leave Nobody but the Baby"
Go to sleep, you little baby
(Go to sleep, you little babe)
Go to sleep, you little baby

(Go to sleep, you little babe)
Your mama's gone away and your daddy's gonna stay
Didn't leave nobody but the baby
Go to sleep, you little baby
(Go to sleep, you little babe)
Go to sleep, you little baby
(Go to sleep, you little babe)
Everybody's gone in the cotton and the corn
Didn't leave nobody but the baby
You're a sweet little baby
(You're a sweet little babe)
You're a sweet little baby
(You're a sweet little babe)
Honey in the rock and the sugar don't stop
Gonna bring a bottle to the baby
Don't you weep, pretty baby
(Don't you weep, pretty babe)
Don't you weep, pretty baby
(Don't you weep, pretty babe)
She's long gone with her red shoes on
Gonna need another lovin' baby

"Stay Awake"

Stay awake, don't rest your head
Don't lie down upon your bed
While the moon drifts in the skies
Stay awake, don't close your eyes
Though the world is fast asleep
Though your pillow soft and deep
You're not sleepy as you seem

Stay awake, don't nod and dream
Stay awake, don't nod and dream

"Lullaby and Goodnight" (Brahms' lullaby)
"Beddy - Bye Butterfly"
"Simple Gifts"
"Danny Boy"
"When You Wish Upon a Star"
"The Rainbow Connection"
"All the Pretty Little Ponies"
"Twinkle, Twinkle, Little Star"
"Beautiful Dreamer"
"Too Ra Loo Ra Loo Ral (That's an Irish Lullaby)"
"Edelweiss"
"All Through the Night"
"Sleep, Baby Sleep"
"All I have to Do Is Dream"
"Hushabye Mountain"
"Swing Low, Sweet Chariot"
"Que Sera, Sera (Whatever Will Be, Will Be)"
"It's you I like"
"Silent Night"
"My Bonnie Lies Over the Ocean"
"I Want to Hold Your Hand"
"La La Lu"
"Puff the Magic Dragon"
"Your Song"
"Count Your Blessings (Instead of Sheep)
"My Favorite Things"
"Star Light, Star Bright"

"Lullabye (Goodnight, My Angel)"
"Baby Mine"
"Sweet Dreams (Goodnight Song)"
"Kumbaya"
"Count Your Blessings Instead of Sheep"
"It's Raining, It's Pouring"
"What a Wonderful World"
"Stand by Me"

38

Tongue twisters

There's nothing quite like a good ole's tongue twister to get you and the kids all caught up in giggles.

These great little poems are full of tongue tangling words that are lots of fun to learn.

They challenge your brain to get the rhythm and the words just right.

You have to take your time with these phrases of alliterative words that sound so much alike can be a real challenge.

Very often children have problems pronouncing certain sounds. The same grandmother's tales and nursery rhymes will help here. They'll go a long way in helping your little ones develop verbal skills. Tongue twisters challenge their little minds in developing strong memory skills, pronunciation and mental reasoning.

Tongue twisters can range from just a single sentence to a whole poem. Here are some great tongue tangling rhymes for you and your special little ones to enjoy.

Go ahead and take up the challenge!

Learn something new, have a few laughs, have contests to see who can get the furthest through the poem without getting all tongue tied!

Check out the list of tongue twisters to get you started!

<h1 style="text-align:center">39</h1>

In order to learn to pronounce b, p, v, f, g, k, d, t,

Betty Botter
Betty Botter bought some butter,
But she said,"The butter's bitter.
If I put it in my batter,
It will make my batter bitter;
But a bit of better butter,
That would make my batter better."
So she bought a bit of butter
Better than her bitter butter,
And she put it in her batter
And the batter was not bitter.
So 'twas better Betty Botter
Bought a bit of better butter.

Billy Button
Billy Button bought a buttered biscuit,
Did Billy Button buy buttered biscuit?

If Billy Button bought a buttered biscuit,
Where's the buttered biscuit Billy Button bought?

Betty the Bee

Betty the Bee has a beautiful buzz.
She bumbles along through the blue skies above.
She breezes by birds and a boisterous bunny
To find a bouquet that will help her make honey!

Pheasant Plucker

I am not a pheasant plucker,
I'm a pheasant plucker's son,
But I'll be plucking pheasants,
When the pheasant plucker's gone.

I Wish To Wish

I wish to wish the wish you wish,
But if you wish the wish the witch wishes,
I won't wish the wish you wish to wish.

Weather Be Fine

Whether the weather be fine,
Or whether the weather be not;
Whether the weather be cold,
Or whether the weather be hot;
We'll weather the weather
Whether we like it or not!

Wood Turtle

How much myrtle would a wood turtle hurdle
If a wood turtle could hurdle myrtle?
A wood turtle would hurldle as much myrtle
As a wood turtle could hurdle
If a wood turtle could hurdle myrtle.

How Much Wood
Woodchuck

How much wood would a woodchuck chuck,
If a woodchuck could chuck wood?
A woodchuck would chuck as much wood,
As a woodchuck would chuck,
If a woodchuck could chuck wood.

Esau Sawed Wood

Esau Wood sawed wood,
All the wood Esau saw,
Esau Wood would saw;
All the wood Wood saw,
Esau sought to saw.
One day Esau Wood's wood-saw would saw no wood,
So Esau Wood sought a new wood-saw;
The new wood-saw would saw wood,
Oh, the wood Esau Wood would saw.
Esau sought a saw that would saw wood
As no other wood-saw would saw.
And Esau found a saw that would saw
As no other wood-saw would saw,

And Esau sawed wood.

One One

One-One was a racehorse,
Two-Two was one, too!
When One-One won one race,
Two-Two won one too!
On mules we find two legs behind
And two we find before.
We stand behind before we find
What those behind be for!

Faith the Fish

Faith the Fish is fantastically fond
Of the frogs and flamingos that live in her pond
They bring ferns and fresh flowers for their fishy friend
And plant them in fans by the waterfall's end.

Fellow

Once a fellow met a fellow
In a field of beans,
Said a fellow to a fellow
"If a fellow asks a fellow,
Can a fellow tell a fellow
What a fellow means?"

Felt

Of all the felt I ever felt,
I never felt a piece of felt,
Which felt as fine as that felt felt,
When first I felt that felt hat's felt.

Freaky Fred

If Freaky Fred found fifty feet of fruit,
And fed forty feet to his friend Frank,
How many feet of fruit did Freaky Fred find?

Fuzzy Wuzzy

Fuzzy Wuzzy was a bear,
Fuzzy Wuzzy had no hair,
So, Fuzzy Wuzzy wasn't really fuzzy,
Was he?

Mr Fister

There once was man who had a sister,
His name was Mr. Fister;
Mr. Fister's sister sold sea shells by the sea shore,
Mr. Fister didn't sell sea shells,
He sold silk sheets,
Mr. Fister told his sister,
That he sold silk six silk sheets to six sheiks;
The sister of Mr. Fister said,
I sold six shells to six sheiks too!

A Flea and A Fly
A flea and a fly,
Flew up in a flue.
Said the flea, "Let us fly!"
Said the fly, "Let us flee!"
So they flew through a flap in the flue.

Groundhog Grind
How much ground would a groundhog grind,
If a groundhog could grind ground?
A groundhog would grind all the ground,
If a groundhog could grind ground.

Grace the Goat
Grace the Goat likes to go very far
Through the gate to get grapes and to play her guitar
She gets gloves as a gift for her friend the gorilla:
They play games wiith goose and green caterpillar.

Can A Canner Can
How many cans can a canner can,
If a canner can can cans?
A canner can can as many cans as a canner can can,
If a canner can can cans.

Cathy the Cat
Cathy the cat is a cuddle creature

And constantly combing her coat keeps it cleaner.
She creeps by a cactus and little toy camel
To carry her cupcake up into her castle.

Dewdrop

How much dew does a dewdrop drop
If dewdrops do drop dew?
They do drop, they do
As do dewdrops drop
If dewdrops do drop dew.

Doctor Another Doctor

If one doctor doctors another doctor,
Does the doctor who doctors the doctor,
Doctor the way the doctor he is doctoring doctor?
Or does he doctor the doctor,
The way the doctor who doctors doctor?

Danielle the Dog

Danielle the Dog likes to dance all day long
While her buddy the duck drums along with a song
When they're done, they get donuts and turn out the light
Dreaming dreams about diamonds and dragons all night.

Theophilus Thaddeus Thistledown

Theophilus Thadeus Thistledown,
The successful thistle-sifter,

While sifting a sieve full of unsifted thistles,
Thrust three thousand thistles
Through the thick of his thumb.
Now, if Theophilus Thadeus Thistledown,
The successfu thistle-sifter,
Thrust three thousand thistles
Through the thick of his thumb,
See that thou,
While sifting a sieve full of unsifted thistles,
Thrust not three thousand thistles
Through the thick of my thumb.

Thought A Thought
I thought a thought,
But the thought I thought
Wasn't the thought I thought i thought;
If the thought I thought
Had been the thought I thought,
I wouldn't have thought so much.

Tree Toad
A tree toad loved a she toad,
Who lived up in a tree,
He was a two-toed tree toad,
But a three-toed toad was she.
The two-toed tree toad tried to win,
The three-toed she toad's heart,
For the two-toed tree toad loved the ground,
That the three-toed tree toad trod.

But the two toed tree toad trod tried in vain,
He couldn't please her whim,
From her tree toad bower,
With her three-toed power,
The she toad vetoed him.

Tutor

A tutor who tooted the flute,
Tried to tutor two tooters to toot.
Said the two to the tutor,
"Is it tougher to toot
Or to tutor two tooters to toot?"

Twister of Twists

A twister of twists once twisted a twist,
And the twist that he twisted was a three-twisted twist;
Now in twisting this twist,
If a twist should untwist,
Would the twist that untwisted untwist the twists?

40

In order to learn to pronounce r, l, m,n

Robert Rowley
    Robert Rowley rolled a round roll 'round,
    A round roll Robert Rowley rolled 'round,
If Robert Rowley rolled a round roll 'roundm
Where rolled the round roll Robert Rowley rolled 'round?

Light A Night Light
You've no need to light a night light
On a light night like tonight,
For a night light's light's a slight light,
And tonight's a night that's light.
When a night's light, like tonight's light,
It is really not quite right
To light a night lights with their slight lights,
On a light night like tonight.

Love's A Feeling

Love's a feeling you feel
When you feel
You're going to feel the feeling
You've never felt before.

Luke Luck

Luke Luck likes lakes,
Luke's duck likes lakes,
Luke Luck licks lakes,
Luke's duck licks lakes,
Duck takes licks in lakes Luke Luck likes,
Luke Luck takes licks in lakes duck likes.

Moses Supposes

Moses supposes his toeses are roses,
But Moses supposes erroneously;
For nobody's toeses are posies or roses,
As Moses supposes his toeses to be.

Millicent

The bottle of perfume that Willy sent
Was highly displeasing to Millicent;
Her thanks so cold
That they quarreled I'm told
O'er that silly scent Willy sent to Millicent.

Mr See Owned A Saw

Mr. See owned a saw,

And Mr. soar owned a seesaw,

Now See's saw sawed Mr. Soar's seesaw,

Before Soar saw See;

Which made Soar sore.

Had Soar seen See's saw,

See's saw would not have sawed Soar's seesaw,

So See's saw sawed Soar's seesaw,

But it was sad to see Soar so sore,

Just because See's saw sawed

Soar's seesaw!

Mr Fister

There once was man who had a sister,

His name was Mr. Fister;

Mr. Fister's sister sold sea shells by the sea shore,

Mr. Fister didn't sell sea shells,

He sold silk sheets,

Mr. Fister told his sister,

That he sold silk six silk sheets to six sheiks;

The sister of Mr. Fister said,

I sold six shells to six sheiks too!

Nobody

This is story about four people named Everybody,

Somebody, Anybody and Nobody,

There was an important job to be done

And Everybody was sure that Somebody would do it,

Anybody could have done it,

But Nobody did it;
Somebody got angry about that,
Because it was Everybody's job,
Everybody thought Anybody could do it,
But Nobody realized that
Everybody wouldn't do it,
It ended up that Everybody
Blamed Somebody,
When Nobody did,
What Anybody could have done.

Ned Nott and Sam Shott

Ned Nott was shot and Sam Shott was not,
So it is better to be Shott than Nott,
Some say Nott was not shot,
But Shott says he shot Nott,
Either the shot Shott shot at Nott was not shot,
Or Nott was shot.
If the shot Shott shot shot Nott,
Nott was shot.
But if the shot Shott shot shot Shott,
Then Shott was shot, not Nott.
However, the shot Shott shot shot not Shott, but Nott!

41

In order to learn to pronounce s, sh

Mr Fister

There once was man who had a sister,
His name was Mr. Fister;
Mr. Fister's sister sold sea shells by the sea shore,
Mr. Fister didn't sell sea shells,
He sold silk sheets,
Mr. Fister told his sister,
That he sold silk six silk sheets to six sheiks;
The sister of Mr. Fister said,
I sold six shells to six sheiks too!

Susan Shineth

Susan shineth shoes and socks,
Socks and shoes shines Susan.
She ceased shining shoes and socks,
For shoes and socks shock Susan!

Mr See Owned A Saw

Mr. See owned a saw,
And Mr. soar owned a seesaw,
Now See's saw sawed Mr. Soar's seesaw,
Before Soar saw See;
Which made Soar sore.
Had Soar seen See's saw,
See's saw would not have sawed Soar's seesaw,
So See's saw sawed Soar's seesaw,
But it was sad to see Soar so sore,
Just because See's saw sawed
Soar's seesaw!

Ned Nott and Sam Shott

Ned Nott was shot and Sam Shott was not,
So it is better to be Shott than Nott,
Some say Nott was not shot,
But Shott says he shot Nott,
Either the shot Shott shot at Nott was not shot,
Or Nott was shot.
If the shot Shott shot shot Nott,
Nott was shot.
But if the shot Shott shot shot Shott,
Then Shott was shot, not Nott.
However, the shot Shott shot shot not Shott, but Nott!

Swan Swam Over The Sea

Swan swam over the sea,
Swim, swam, swim!

Swan swim back again,
Well swum, swan!

A Sailor Went To Sea

A sailor went to sea, sea, sea,
To see what he could see, see, see,
And all that he could see, see, see,
Was the bottom of the deep blue sea, sea, sea.

Surely Sylvia Swims

Surely Sylvia swims shrieked Sammy,
Someone should show Sylvia some strokes
So she shall not sink!

I Slit A Sheet

I slit a sheet,
A sheet I slit,
And on a slitted sheet I sit.
I slit a sheet,
A sheet I slit,
The sheet I slit,
That sheet was it.

Swiss Witches

Three switched Swiss witches,
Watch three washed Swiss witch,
Swatch watch switches,

Which sweet switched Swiss witch watches,
Which washed Swiss witch,
Swatch watch switch!

Sheila Shorter

Sheila Shorter sought a suitor,
Sheila sought a suitor short,
Sheila's suitor's sure to suit her
Short's the suitor Sheila sought!

Skunk On A Stump

A skunk sat on a stump,
The stump thought the skunk stunk,
The skunk thought the stump stunk,
What stunk, the skunk or the stump?

See's Saw

Mr. See owned a saw,
And Mr. Soar owned a seesaw,
Now See's saw sawed Mr. Soar's seesaw,
Before Soar saw See,
Which made Soar sore.
Had Soar seen See's saw,
See's saw would not have sawed Soar's seesaw,
So See's saw sawed Soar's seesaw,
But it was sad to see Soar's so sore,
Just because See's saw sawed,
Soar's seesaw!

She Sells Seashells

She sells sea shells on the sea shore,
The shells that she sells are sea shells,
I'm sure.
So if she sells sea shells
on the sea shore,
I'm sure that the shells are
sea shore shells.

Silly Sally

Silly Sally shooed seven silly sheep,
The seven silly sheep silly Sally shooed,
Shilly- sallied south.
These sheep shouldn't sleep in a shack,
Sheep should sleep in a shed.

42

In order to learn to pronounce other sounds…

Hottentot
    If a Hottentot taught a Hottentot tot
    To talk 'ere the tot could totter,
Ought the Hottentot tot
Be taught to say aught or naught,
Or what ought to be taught her?
If to hoot and to toot a Hottentot tot
Be taught by her Hottentot tutor,
Ought the tutor get hot
If the Hottentot tot
Hoot and toot at her Hottentot tutor?

Elizabeth the Elephant
Elizabeth the Elephant escaped from the zoo
And the elk and the eagle escaped with her, too
But an elephant eats an enormous amount:
Too many enchiladas, and eggplant, and egg rollsto count.

Understand

If you understand, say "understand"
If you don't understand, say "don't understand"
But if you understand and say "don't understand"
How do I understand that you understand?
Understand?

Yellow Butter, Purple Jelly

Yellow butter, purple jelly, red jam, black bread,
Spread it thick, say it quick,
Yellow butter, purple jelly, red jam, black bread,
Spread it thicker, say it quick,
Yellow butter, purple jelly, red jam, black bread,
Don't eat with your mouth full.

April the Alligator

April the Alligator is always awake
Swimming round and round her aquarium lake
Adding apples and airplanes and ants in her head.
Close your eyes, April!
Away to your bed.

43

Resources

Vengrow, B. (2024, January 2). *Introducing tummy time to baby.* https://www.thebump.com/a/tummy-time-when-to-start-how-to-do

Stanford, K. (2023, December 28). *10 weird (but totally normal) things about your newborn.* https://www.thebump.com/a/10-totally-weird-but-totally-normal-things-about-your-newborn

Charaipotra, S. (2020, March 3). *Tips for how to get baby to sleep.* https://www.thebump.com/a/helping-baby-sleep-better

If you found this book helpful, I'd be very appreciative if you left a favorable review for the book on Amazon!